# Healing Inflammatory Bowel Disease

## The Cause and Cure of Crohn's Disease and Ulcerative Colitis

Answers to Questions about IBD
by a Former Sufferer Healed
through Nature's Cure

*Dear Florence*
*YHWA Bless You!*

## Paul Nison

Layout and design: Kira Knight

Cover design: Kira Knight and Paul Nison

Editor: Joel Brody

Library of Congress Catalog Card Number:

ISBN#: 0-9675286-3-1

343 Publishing Company
P.O. Box 16156
West Palm Beach, FL 33416

# Acknowledgements

First, I have to acknowledge God. Without God, life is meaningless.

Everyone I've met over the years has helped me to heal myself of IBD and has supported me and kept me healthy. When I think about IBD and my personal victory over it, I want to give special acknowledgement to the following people:

Brian Clement and The Hippocrates Health Institute in West Palm Beach, Florida.

All the great people over the years at The Accent on Wellness support group in New York City: Tom Coviello, Matthew Grace, Donna Perrone and Ed Lieb.

All the people who helped me with the raw diet when I was first stating out: Roe Gallo, David Wolfe, Thor Blazor, David Klein, Morris Krok, and Ana Vicenti.

And all the people over the years who helped and supported me, Far too many people to name, but you know who you are. And most of all, Dr. Fred Bisci who has taught me more about the human body, the spiritual body, and the mental aspects of health than anyone else.

For encouraging me to write this book, I want to acknowledge everyone who has asked my advice about IBD over the years.

For their support and help in getting this book done: Joel Brody and Kira Knight.

Finally, certain sections presented in this book were based on information I've learned from the many books I've read over the years on the subject of intestinal health. I thank the authors and publishers of all those books for their contribution to helping people realize that nutrition can be an important factor when dealing with IBD. Though I don't agree 100% with all the books out there on the subject of IBD, all the books I've read have some excellent insight to help people overcome IBD, as well as many other diseases. To all authors on the subject of IBD, thank you so much for helping me and so many others. May God bless you for your humane work.

# Dedication

This book is dedicated to everyone who has suffered from any so-called "incurable" disease. There are no incurable diseases, only incurable thinking. Keep looking for the answers, and you will find them. God bless you.

# Contents

# Foreword

Dr. Fred Bisci

The subject of health and healing in today's society has led to much confusion. There is a prolific amount of information, alternative ideas and so-called experts who are all extolling varied ideas. The sheer flood of information at hand leaves the average person perplexed.

In my almost forty years of involvement with health and nutrition and as a nutritional consultant, I've met some people who really left an impact and made a difference. Paul Nison is one of those people.

The first time I met Paul was when he came to my office to interview me for his first book. Since that time, I have watched Paul become a popular author and profound public speaker. He travels the world determined to bring his message about health and raw foods in a manner that few have done. His energy and vibrancy have been equaled by few. Having traveled with him myself, it has been a joy to observe his enthusiasm in reaching as many people as he can and continuing to search and learn along the way. In this book that Paul has written on inflammatory bowel disease, I see that he once again reflects on health in a way that is simple, yet very profound. Paul has a unique way of sharing his experience in a clear and precise manner. Paul has an understanding that the human body has a God-given remedial ability to heal itself from disease, if the causes of disease are omitted or removed.

In this book, Paul tells his story about his journey and his experience of how he healed himself from a serious case of ulcerative colitis. He understands that we, as natural beings, are subject to all of the rules of natural law and cannot avoid the problems we create by a perversion of a healthy dietary lifestyle. He gives mystifying concepts clarity, and therefore delivers them to the consciousness of the average individual. Paul understands the connection that links emotions, spirituality and the human body's fine-tuned functions.

Having worked with numerous cases of people who have suffered from inflammatory bowel disease, watching them change their lifestyle and seeing their bodies heal themselves, I would recommend Paul's book with enthusiasm to any person that is suffering from ulcerative colitis or Crohn's disease. I think that Paul has done it again by writing another book that everyone will enjoy reading and will be of benefit to anyone who has a similar problem.

Fred Bisci,
Ph.D., N.C

# Introduction

*How did you cure yourself of inflammatory bowel disease?*

That's the question people suffering with IBD ask me all the time. According to doctors, it's an incurable disease. After explaining how I did cure myself to so many people, many tried my suggestions and got better. As more people got better, they would tell someone they knew who was sick, and many more people would come to me and ask, "How did you do it?" or, even more often, "How can I do it?" Finally, I decided the best way to convey this information with my answers is to write a book.

When I decided to write this book, I wanted to have a book that people could easily understand and get results immediately upon following my advice. For this to happen, they would have to be motivated to read the book. I've read many books on IBD, and most of them begin by giving information about the digestive organs: what they are, where they are, and how they work. I admit it can be quite interesting and educational to learn about this, but a sick person wants results as fast as possible. I believe this is not the time to give a physiology lesson. In my opinion, that would only confuse readers — increasing the risk of their not finishing the book and having to look elsewhere for the answers. Although such physiological information is educational, for the sake of the sufferers, I've decided to leave such information out of this book. I suffered from IBD for years and understand how you feel if you're also suffering from it. I'm not a doctor writing a book, but a person who has suffered with IBD for many years before finding the answers that enabled me to heal. I understand what you're going through. I know your mindset and your fears.

If you want to learn about the physiology of the human body, most other books on the subject of IBD or intestinal disease would have this information, as would a medical dictionary or physiology book. Instead, in this book, I decided to focus on two major issues: the cause of IBD and the natural cure for IBD. When I was sick, all I could think of while suffering was: "I don't care what it's called, how it looks, why I have it, just tell me how to get rid of it." If I see one more picture of a normal colon and one with IBD, I'll go crazy. That's why I've decided not to put many pictures or graphics in this book.

Another problem I found was that many books talk about how to live with IBD since the authors don't know of a cure. I would rather focus on how to get rid of IBD as soon as possible without ever getting used to living with it. You don't have to get used to it because you can get rid of it.

Unlike anything you may have heard, there is much information now to prove IBD is a dietary disease and also stress related. Making a few dietary improvements, such as replacing the low quality food in your diet with higher quality food, along with reducing the stress in your life, can be the difference between sickness and cure. In this book, I focus mostly on how to improve your diet. I also explain other important factors to keep you healthy once you are cured. In the future, I plan to write an extensive book on the issue of reducing stress, dealing with emotional/spiritual aspects of health and healing.

# Part One:

## My Interest in Inflammatory Bowel Disease

Until age nineteen, I ate the standard American diet (also known as the S.A.D diet, and it is very SAD) and never suffered from any problems other than the common upset stomach or headache. Sometimes I would get a cold, but I thought that was normal. But, then, the stomachaches started to get worse. I would get colds more often, and I started to worry. I decided to go to the hospital and get checked to see what the problem was. After I was subjected to the doctors' many tests, they told me I had food poisoning. They gave me some medication and sent me home. I thought the drugs the doctors gave me would cure me, but during the following three weeks the pains kept coming back worse and worse. They got so bad that many times I wasn't even able to walk five feet without having to go to the bathroom, whether I had eaten or not. I was wasting away. My weight dropped to 125 pounds, and everyone I knew told me I looked terrible. I tried everything I could think of that would put weight on my body. I ate big portions of fatty foods with increasing frequency. Plus, I stopped doing all exercise in order not to burn too many calories. Nothing I tried worked; my condition just kept getting worse. I was willing to deal with the intense pain, but then one night, I saw blood in my stool. Now, I was really scared. I went to the doctor, and the lab ran many tests on me. I felt like some scientific experiment. But, I would have done anything to find out what the problem was, so it could be cured. Up until then, I thought everyone had the common pain I was having. But once

I saw blood, I knew the problem was much more serious than I had ever imagined.

Finally, from the doctor, I received my wake-up call. I was diagnosed with inflammatory bowel disease. It was so bad, the doctor didn't know if it was ulcerative colitis or Crohn's and said it might even be both.

Although most people would consider this a tragedy, as I also did at that time, now I consider it one of the best things that ever happened to me. When I found out what I had, I remember thinking to myself, "Now I can stop trying to figure out what the problem is and let the doctors cure me." What a big mistake that was.

The doctors, or the drugs the doctors gave me, did not work. In fact, to this day, with all the technology doctors have, there is still no known medical cure for ulcerative colitis or Crohn's disease. The only natural relief from the pain for most people, as it was for me, is to go to the bathroom very often and sit there for about thirty minutes to an hour. I remember when I was in the bathroom, no matter where it was, people would knock on the door and ask me if I was okay. I would think, "NO, I'm not okay, I'm very sick," but I never said anything because who would understand? How many people ever heard of ulcerative colitis or knew what it was? In brief, for those of you who still don't understand what it is, ulcerative colitis or Crohn's disease is not an easy illness to live with. The colon is achy and inflamed. With UC there are many ulcerations, often with bleeding. It's accompanied by spasmodic and frequent bowel movements. The typically poor diet, increased bowel movements, decreased assimilation of swallowed food, and along with drug therapies, all add up to malnutrition, decreased vitality, stress, emotional unhappiness, not to mention misery and a ruined life.

I would get colitis flare-ups many times throughout the year. Every time I went to the doctor, she told me to stay away from dairy foods until I felt better. Then, she increased the dosage of steroids she was giving me. After a few weeks, when I would feel better, she said it was okay to eat dairy foods again. I would then eat foods that contained huge amounts of dairy. Sometimes this would be a whole big pizza. Then the flare-ups came back. Finally, I recognized the pattern and cut out dairy products altogether. I was very pleased with the results. I got sick less often. After that, I began to eliminate whatever the doctors told me was okay to eat: eggs, meat and sugar to name just a few. I told my doctor, "I feel better without these foods."

She told me, "Food has nothing to do with your condition." After hearing that from her, I knew I was on the right track. I said to myself, "If she's such a good doctor, why do I keep seeing the same people in the waiting room every time I come for a visit? She doesn't heal them, that's why. If she did, they wouldn't need to come back."

At age twenty-three, I left my stressful job as an office manager for a big Wall Street firm in New York's financial district and moved to West Palm Beach, Florida. I was still having colitis flare-ups, but not as often or severe. By seemingly sheer coincidence, I moved near a place called the Hippocrates Health Institute. I would visit the Institute often during my daily walks around the neighborhood. It was there that I learned about the raw-food lifestyle and about live foods. I immediately put myself on an 80% raw-food diet. What a difference it made! I told my doctor in New York about my improvement, and she said, "Raw foods are no good for your condition." Once again, I knew I was on the right track!

Here's where the doctors made the mistake: raw foods were not as much the problem as was eating them in their whole form. When a person is suffering from IBD, whole foods can cause problems, however, eating raw foods in their blended form was the answer I needed. Medical doctors have not been trained in the benefits of eating blended salads and vegetable juices. The key I found was to give the body the nourishment it needs, but at the same time, rest is also needed to heal. A diet of fresh raw juices and blended foods, in my opinion, is the answer. Not just for me, this program works for EVERYONE who does it correctly.

Since adopting the raw-food diet, I've gone through several "healing crises." I'm happy for these episodes of elimination, as they are clearly my body's way of cleaning, healing and rejuvenating. At one point, my weight went all the way down to 118 pounds, but, by then, I had gained an understanding of how the body works, and I didn't panic. Now my weight remains at a healthy looking 145 pounds, and I know the raw-food diet is the best way for me to go.

Since going 100% raw, I have completely overcome IBD. I can now eat raw foods in their whole form with no problems, and I feel better than ever. I have also become increasingly inspired about life.

I was so amazed with my results, I tried to explain the vast improvement in my health to my doctor and others, but they all told me I was wrong, or I was one in a million. They told me raw foods couldn't cure colitis or anything else. After talking to many people about it, I began to believe that I was wasting my time. No one wanted to listen to me. So I decided not to talk about it anymore. I knew I was cured and feeling better. That was the only important thing for me at that time in my life.

I never wanted to talk about my healing after that until my good friend, who I hadn't seen in a while, called to inform me that he had recently been diagnosed with ulcerative colitis.

At first, I was hesitant to talk to him about it. But after hearing about the pain he was going through and understanding it, I felt I had to. I told him my story and everything I went through, and how I got better. He seemed very wary of giving it a try because his doctor had told him, "Raw foods are bad for someone with ulcerative colitis." After telling him the doctors told me the same thing, he said he would give it a try. I advised him to go on a fresh fruit juice diet for 24 hours. He said he knew what fresh juices were, and I made the mistake of assuming he did — big error on my part.

On the following day, his mother called screaming at me that I tried to kill her son. I asked what the problem was, and she told me he had to be rushed to the hospital.

He called me a few days later, and when I asked him what the problem was, he told me my suggestion didn't work and made his condition worse. I asked him what juice he'd used. He told me Gatorade, a sports drink. I told him that wasn't a fresh juice, and he told me that the doctors told him it was the worst case of a UC attack they had ever seen. (I've heard this many times from many UC sufferers.) To make matters worse, the hospital was feeding him very unhealthy food.

The final result was my friend decided to go through with the operation and get his colon taken out. He just hadn't found an answer and wasn't willing to live with the pain. I can relate to not wanting to live with the pain. After hearing his story, I decided I must provide people with information about the raw food diet and health. People need to know that there is, in fact, a way to heal naturally. It is a fact that if you eliminate the cause, you will eliminate the problem.

Exhibits from the author's medical records

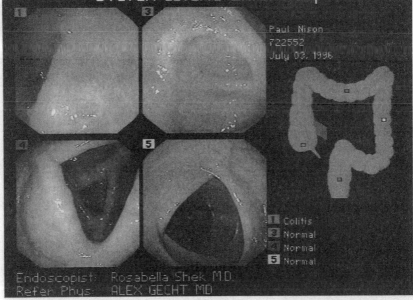

```
                                   Staten Island University Hospital                    PAGE 1
RUN ON 07/05/96-1711    475 SEAVIEW AVE SIGNED OUT REPORT           RUN FOR 07/05/96
                                         SHEK, ROSABELLA MD


PATIENT NAME:        NISON,PAUL                          LOCATION: AMBULATORY SURGERY
=============================================================================================
**96:S0008767U **    A/C:05791833   U:(000722552  )   25 M                    AMBULREG
===================

                 COLL:07/03/96  UNK  RECV:07/03/96 0829   SHEK, ROSABELLA MD
```

CLINICAL HISTORY
    INDICATION(S) FOR PROCEDURE(S): Ulcerative colitis
    PRE-OP  DX: Same
    POST-OP DX: Same

SURGICAL PROCEDURE

  COLONOSCOPY

SPECIMEN

  A) Right colon
  B) Transverse colon
  C) Left colon
  D) Rectum

GROSS DESCRIPTION

  A) The specimen is labeled "right colon". The specimen, sent in formalin,
consists of three fragments of grayish tissue each 2 mm in diameter,
submitted entirely as a rush.                     (1 block)

  B) The specimen is labeled "transverse". The specimen, sent in formalin,
consists of two fragments of grayish tissue each 2 mm in diameter,
submitted entirely as a rush.                     (1 block)

  C) The specimen is labeled "left colon". The specimen, sent in formalin,
consists of two fragments of grayish tissue each 2 mm in diameter,
submitted entirely as a rush.                     (1 block)

  D) The specimen is labeled "rectal". The specimen, sent in formalin,
consists of two fragments of grayish tissue each 2 mm in diameter,
submitted entirely as a rush.                     (1 block)
    Dictated By: KAHNG,H  M.D.

    * * * F I N A L   D I A G N O S I S * * *

A)B)C)D)  MUCOSAL ULCERATIVE COLITIS, MOST SEVERE IN THE RECTUM AND MILD
    IN OTHER SITES.


Signed-out: KAHNG,H  M.D.                  _____  07/05/96
```

RECEIVED
JUL 12 1996
```

```
        STATEN ISLAND        9.10    PATIENT NAME: NISON, PAUL
     UNIVERSITY HOSPITAL
     475   SEAVIEW AVENUE            MEDICAL RECORD NO:   722552
  STATEN ISLAND, NEW YORK 10305
                                     DATE OF OPERATION:   09/10/93
     REPORT OF OPERATION
```

SURGEON:                        ROSABELLA SHEK, M.D.

ASSISTANT SURGEON:

ANESTHESIA:

PREOPERATIVE DIAGNOSIS:

POSTOPERATIVE DIAGNOSIS:

OPERATION PERFORMED:        COLONOSCOPY
                            BIOPSY

INDICATIONS:
The patient  is a 22 year old male with a history of ulcerative
colitis and continual rectal bleeding depsite Rowasa enema
therapy.

PROCEDURE:
The patient was placed in the left lateral decubitus position,
conscious sedation was given with Demerol and Valium. Complete
evaluation was remarkable for excessive edema, erythema with
punctate superficial erosions throughout the entire ascending and
transverse colon.  Biopsy of this area was taken.

The descending colon was relatively normal except for some
localized areas of a few superficial erosions with minimal
erythema or edema.  The rectum and sigmoid was moderately involved
to the anal verge with erythematous and edematous folds and loss
of mucosal architecture and superficial erosions.  Biopsy of this
area was taken.  Photographs of the involved areas were taken. The
endoscope was withdrawn. The patient tolerated the procedure well.
The patient was transferred to the Recovery Room in a stable
condition.

IMPRESSION:
The minimal involvement of the descending colon may be related
to response to enema therapy. However given the spotty involvement
of the descending colon and consideration of Crohn's disease
rather than ulcerative colitis needs to be entertained at this
time.

**MetPath**

Teterboro Laboratory
One Malcolm Avenue
Teterboro, New Jersey 0~ ~-1070
201-393-5000
800-631-1390 Client Service

**Clinical
Laboratory
Report**

RAYMOND GAMBINO, M.D.
PAUL A. KRIEGER M.D.
JOSEPH E. O'BRIEN, M.D.
CHARLENE S. POLAN, M.D.

| Patient Name | | Date Drawn | | Date Received | Date of Report |
|---|---|---|---|---|---|
| NISON, PAUL | 00503 | 04/13/93 | | 04/13/93 | 04/16/93 |

| Sex | Age | | Client Name / Address | | I.D. Number | Account Number |
|---|---|---|---|---|---|---|
| M | 23 | 1A | STATEN ISLAND F. P. | 1A | | 56711 |

Referring Physician: SHEK
3HN064660

45 MC CLEAN AVENUE
STATEN ISLAND NY 10306

C.L.I.A. #31D0696246
Specimen Number: L35085
Time Draw

Patient I.D./Soc. Sec Number

TISSUE PATHOLOGY -

GROSS FINDINGS - THE SPECIMEN CONSISTS OF TWO PIECES OF TISSUE, EACH
MEASURING APPROXIMATELY, IN CM., 0.3X0.2X0.1 THE ENTIRE SPECIMEN IS
SUBMITTED FOR SECTIONING. THE NUMBER OF CASSETTES PROCESSED IS ONE. THE
SPECIMEN CONTAINER IS LABELLED WITH THE PATIENT'S NAME.

MICROSCOPIC DIAGNOSIS - FRAGMENTS OF COLONIC MUCOSA WITH ACUTE AND CHRONIC
INFLAMMATION, CRYPT ABSCESSES AND SURFACE EROSIONS. BIOPSIES FROM RECTUM.

NOTE- THE FINDINGS ARE CONSISTENT WITH CHRONIC IDIOPATHIC INFLAMMATORY
BOWEL DISEASE, FAVOR ULCERATIVE COLITIS.

DIAGNOSED BY

DUSAN TISMA, M. D.

NXC/DXT/4

---

NAME: NISON, PAUL
TYPE OF REPORT: OPERATIVE REPORT

M.R. NO. 722552
DATE:     09/10/93

PAGE: 2

PLAN:
1. Folow up on biopsy results
2. Start Asacol 800 mg t.i.d.
3. Prednisone 20 mg daily
4. The patient will see me in the office in one week

ROSABELLA SHEK, M.D.

Dictated by: Rosabella Shek, M.D.

RS/stl/RR
D: 09/10/93
T: 09/13/93
TAPE#: 6844
JOB#:  0133
913NSI1.STL
cc: Rosabella Shek, M.D.

22

# COLONOSCOPY REPORT
STATEN ISLAND UNIVERSITY HOSPITAL ENDOSCOPY UNIT / NORTH DIVISION

**DATE:** July 3, 1996
**ENDOSCOPIST:** Rosabella Shek M.D.
**REFERRING PHYSICIAN:** ALEX GECHT MD
**PATIENT NAME:** Paul Nison
**HOSPITAL NO:** 722552
**HISTORY/INDICATIONS:**
    This colonoscopy was performed for evaluation of history of
    ulcerative colitis.
**INSTRUMENT:** CF-100TL
**MEDICATIONS:**
    Preoperative:      Demerol (meperidine) 50 mg IV
                    Valium (diazepam) 20 mg IV
**BIOPSIES:** yes     **BRUSHINGS:** no     **PHOTOGRAPHS:** yes
**PROCEDURE:**
    A history and physical examination were performed. The procedure,
    indications, potential complications (bleeding, perforation, infection,
    adverse medication reaction), and alternatives available were explained
    to the patient who appeared to understand and indicated this.
    Opportunity for questions was provided and informed consent obtained.
    After placing the patient in the left lateral decubitus position, the
    colonoscope was inserted into the rectum and under direct visualization
    advanced to the cecum which was identified by identification of the
    cecal strap (crow's foot), identification of the appendiceal orifice,
    identification of the ileocecal valve . Careful inspection was made
    as the colonoscope was withdrawn. The quality of the prep was good.
    The patient tolerated the procedure well. There were no complications.
**FINDINGS:**
    - Mucosal changes were noted in the rectum. The findings included an
    erythematous appearance, a friable appearance, a granular appearance,
    petechiae, areas of frank hemorrhage, loss of the interhaustral fold
    pattern, a mucoid discharge. Multiple biopsies were obtained from the
    abnormal mucosa. (Image 1) (Image 3) (Image 4) (Image 5)
    - Other than the findings noted above, the visualized colonic segments
    were normal.
**IMPRESSION:**
    - Mucosal changes (biopsied) compatible with ulcerative colitis
**RECOMMENDATIONS:**
    - Follow-up the biopsy results
    - 5-ASA Enema 1 pr B.I.D.
    - Taper and stop steroids.
    - Lactose - free diet

_____
Rosabella Shek M.D.

# Part Two

## QUESTIONS AND ANSWERS ABOUT IBD YOU NEED TO KNOW

After having read many books on the subject of health, I decided the best style in which to write this book was a question and answer format. Many books put this style in the back of a book, but, as I recall, I always liked that part the best. It answered the most common questions and was right to the point. I have learned that someone going through IBD needs that — someone to get right to the point. As you read these questions and answers, I suggest you keep an open mind and understanding; these will get you the results you are looking for. I have a saying: "Don't deny till you try." If you take my suggestions and don't get the results (which I don't feel will be the case; you will begin to heal by trying my suggestions) then you'll have the right to say, "I've tried it and it didn't work." However, if you never try it, you will never have the right to say you don't believe in it, or it won't work. "Don't deny till you try." You can thank me later, after you're healed. If a doctor tells you that there is no time because it's the worst case he has seen, keep in mind they say this most of the time because that's what they're used to saying. They want to rush you into their way of thinking before you can have a chance to figure it out for yourself. The truth is, if it is that bad and you don't have time, most likely, at that point, the doctors won't be able to help you either. As long as your body is still working and has the energy and function in the organ or diseased body part, it can revert and heal itself naturally.

## What exactly is inflammatory bowel disease, also known as IBD?

Inflammatory bowel disease (IBD), also known as Crohn's disease or ulcerative colitis, is a disease of the gastrointestinal tract. People with ulcerative colitis are only affected in the colon (large intestine), while people with Crohn's disease can be affected in the small intestines or the ileum. There are many other forms of IBD such as, proctitis, enteritis, or ileitis, but Crohn's disease and ulcerative colitis are the most widespread.

In these most widespread forms, the affected areas become inflamed, and sometimes ulceration occurs in the affected areas. When the disease is in its active stage, an inflammation occurs which is commonly referred to as a "flare-up." During an acute inflammation, there occurs what you would expect with any inflammation: swelling, heat, sensitivity to touch, and a lot of pain. When the inflammation continues without stopping, and one or more parts of the intestine is inflamed, much pain is caused along with other problems that will be discussed. Chronic inflammation is a more serious stage that can result in distortion and sometimes destruction of tissues often leading to permanent scarring.

Both Crohn's disease and ulcerative colitis are chronic illnesses according to medical thinking, meaning you will always have them even when they're in remission (inactive).

When the name of a disease ends in "itis," it means there is some form of inflammation involved. All inflammatory diseases are the same; they just occur in different parts of the body. Regardless what part of the body is suffering from inflammation, most likely the problem has the same cause. Depending on what part of the body is affected, some inflammatory diseases can be much more serious than others, but the cause behind them is the same. IBD is a very serious inflammatory disease that, if not taken care of, can lead to still more serious illnesses. There are many very painful inflammatory diseases prevalent today, the most widespread of which is rheumatoid arthritis. However, IBD is the most common. All inflammatory diseases are characterized by periods of inactivity when life is pretty normal, but active periods called flare-ups can make you feel pretty miserable.

## What exactly do you mean by inflamed bowel?

Whenever inflammation is involved, regardless of where in the body it occurs, the tissue has been caused to become inflamed. If the tissue is close to the surface of the body, it can be seen, as in the case of a sprained ankle or some other type of bruise, but if it's deep inside the body, it can still become very inflamed even though you can't see it. An inflamed bowel is similar to any inflamed tissue. A sprain or swollen part of the body such as a bump on the head will hurt when it's touched. An inner swelling, such as arthritis, hurts when the joints are moved.

The bowel is a "tube" deep within the body with a strong outer muscled wall. Inflammation makes its central opening smaller. The open canal of a swollen small intestine can shrink to about an eighth of an inch in diameter, the width of a small drinking straw. Swollen body parts are very tender and need rest. When we sprain an ankle, or get a bump on the head, we don't touch it till it's gone, or the swelling has gone down. Well, when the inside of the body is swollen, we have to try to do the same thing — leave it alone till it's better. When an inflamed intestine is called upon to digest food, it hurts. It becomes very painful, and just as if we were to walk with a sprained ankle, we would slow the healing down and make it worse.

## Once the inflammation goes away, can there still be any damage left behind?

Once the inflammation goes down, or heals, the bowel can return to normal, but when it does, in some cases, deformed scar tissue may remain as a result of the inflammation. This is known as a stricture. It's similar to the deformed scar tissue in an arthritic joint, or the scar tissue left from a serious cut. In the small intestine, the scar tissue can circle the intestine for a short distance in each direction, or it can cover an entire area along the intestine.

A stricture causes trouble because it's an unyielding area in an otherwise homogeneous and smooth organ that undulates in peristaltic motion. Because it's not as flexible, a stricture can't move with the surrounding tissue, so it "pulls" when the intestine moves. Partially digested food can become stuck in a stricture leading to a blockage that can be painful. In severe cases, hospitalization is required to clear the obstruction.

When a stricture is present, hard pieces of food, such as bits of nuts, fruit seeds, or even coarse, undigested bran from cereal, can be irritating.

## Why do some people get less serious forms of inflammatory diseases while others get more serious ones, and still others get none at all?

The body will do it's best to avoid disease, but when the conditions for disease are present and are not dealt with in the right way, we will suffer. Usually, the weakest parts suffer the most or suffer first. That is why not everyone suffers from the same illness. If people don't take care of themselves, they will all suffer from one illness or another. People get different forms of the same diseases. Some people will get arthritis, some will get proctitis, others pancreatits, and still others Crohn's disease or ulcerative colitis. These are all forms of inflammation in some part of the body. The bottom line is there is one cure, and that cure is explained in this book, but first, it is helpful to understand as much about IBD as possible.

## Okay, now I know Crohn's disease and ulcerative colitis are very similar inflammatory diseases, but what are their differences?

There are many similarities between Crohn's disease and ulcerative colitis. Here are the most common differences: ulcerative colitis occurs only in the colon (large intestine) with ulcers, open sores, and inflammation. UC suffers usually have bloody, watery stools with mucus during a flare-up attack. UC can involve different parts of the large intestine, or it can involve the entire organ.

Crohn's disease can affect the small intestines or the ileum, characterized by inflammation that spreads deep into the bowel wall.

One thing that makes them very similar is that there is no known medical cure for IBD, that is unless you consider cutting out the colon as a cure. In that case, there is a cure for UC, but still not for Crohn's. Even so, I don't consider this a cure. This would be like saying there is a cure of colon cancer — cut out the colon, and you can't get cancer.

## Is there a difference between colitis and ulcerative colitis?

There is a difference between colitis and ulcerative colitis. Just as the name states, plain colitis doesn't involve ulcerations and seems to be confined more to the upper part of the large intestine. Ulcerative colitis is a much more serious disease, as you can imagine. Whenever there is ulceration, there is usually blood, and when blood is coming out of the body, it is very serious.

## How serious a disease is IBD?

IBD is very serious. If not taken care of, it can lead to many more problems such as nutrient deficiencies and emotional sickness, all the way to a more serious disease such as colon cancer. Many incidences of IBD can be controlled with drugs, but this can lead to a very painful life unless the illness is cured naturally. The drugs can have some very harmful side effects. IBD is a very serious disease, just as serious as diabetes, cancer, or AIDS.

What are the common symptoms of IBD a person will suffer during an acute stage or an "IBD attack"?

Some common symptoms of IBD that you might experience are pain, poor appetite, flatulence, nausea, diarrhea, and mucus and blood in the stool. Those are the signs you'll notice on your own telling you something is wrong, and there is a chance it might be some form of IBD. There are many other diseases that have the same symptoms as IBD, so if you experience any of these signs, it's just an indication that it could be IBD among other things. Your doctor can perform tests and observe several signs other than how you feel to determine if it's really IBD or something else. (Many times a doctor will misdiagnose IBD at the beginning stages till it gets worse and the signs are more prevalent, but they do have certain tests that they can use to eventually give a correct diagnosis of IBD.) Crohn's disease and ulcerative colitis may have similar symptoms, but may also have different symptoms. The most common sign of UC is bloody diarrhea. It's also possible to have bleeding without diarrhea, and some people even have bleeding with constipation; most of the time though, it's bloody diarrhea. There are other common signs of UC such as a consistent urge to have to go to the bathroom. Many times you get the feeling that you have to go to the bathroom, but, then, when you go, nothing comes out. Sometimes just some gas will come out, or a little blood. Sometimes there is only a very small amount of stool and no blood, but when you wipe, you'll see blood on the toilet paper. With all the false urges and real bowel movements, the number of times you go to the bathroom in one day can get all the way up to twenty. A good indication of the seriousness of the flare-up is how many trips a person with UC takes to the bathroom each day. More trips indicate a more serious flare-up.

The signs for Crohn's disease are very similar to those for UC, and both are often misdiagnosed as the other. With Crohn's, the symptoms can affect the small intestine or the ileum (whereas with UC, it's the large intestine that is affected). The pain is most often felt around the navel and/or lower right part of the abdomen and is often associated with eating. It can begin during a meal, soon after, or within an hour or so afterwards. A steady dull ache in the lower right abdomen may also be felt. It usually becomes somewhat worse with activity, especially anything that jiggles the abdomen, such as jogging. Crohn's patients often suffer from fatigue and poor appetite just as UC sufferers.

### If I have the symptoms you've mentioned, does that mean I have IBD?

Maybe, maybe not. There are many other medical conditions that have similar signs but can be something else. A good doctor, if you can find one, hopefully, will be able to diagnose you correctly. It is common for many people to get diagnosed for another condition before the doctor finally realizes that it's IBD. Conditions that can mimic IBD include food poisoning, traveler's diarrhea, antibiotic use. IBS, or irritable bowel syndrome, can also resemble IBD.

Certain foods can cause diarrhea such as those containing lactose (especially if you're lactose intolerant), as can beverages containing caffeine.

Drugs, including antibiotics and over-the-counter drugs, can cause chronic diarrhea.

Cancer patients get diarrhea from the radiation treatments.

### Other than the common signs, how do I really know if I have IBD?

Other than the many clear symptoms and signs used to find out if a person might have IBD, or other digestive tract problems, the doctor will perform a series of tests to determine if it's IBD or not. The doctor will examine the patient with an endoscope. During the examination of the rectum, the doctor will usually take a biopsy (tissue sample) to confirm the diagnosis. The doctor may also arrange to have the stools sent to a lab to check for infectious diseases that mimic ulcerative colitis. Usually, a patient

31

suspected of having ulcerative colitis will undergo a diagnostic procedure called a sigmoidoscopy which involves passing an instrument (a sigmoidoscope) through the anus into the rectum, and then into the sigmoid colon. This procedure allows the physician to view the mucosa (inner lining) of the bowel. I've had many of these tests performed over the years. My doctor mainly used it to determine the amount of drugs she would give me to control my illness. This is a procedure that can be done in the doctor's office. No hospital visit is required.

A colonoscopy is another diagnostic procedure in which the doctor examines most, or all of the colon. It can be used to diagnose UC, but not Crohn's disease. This procedure will determine how much of the colon is inflamed. During the procedure for some patients, the end of the ileum can also be examined. A colonoscopy can be used to check for colon cancer as well. The procedure is usually done at the hospital, but no overnight visit is necessary.

Crohn's disease is diagnosed with x-rays or other means, but not a colonosopy. This is because most cases of Crohn's disease occur in the ileum, or the ileum and the right side of the colon, and these are areas a colonoscopy won't reach.

It is neither practical nor possible to do a colonoscopy on every person suspected of having the disease. But someone with chronic diarrhea will very likely have a sigmoidoscopy as part of the investigation. In certain cases, when x-rays don't find it, a colonoscopy can be used.

## How come I've never heard of IBD before? Is it a new disease?

You've never heard of IBD before most likely because it affects the colon. Many people are embarrassed to talk about IBD, but it's not a new disease. Both Crohn's disease and ulcerative colitis are very common in today's world and have been around for a long time.

Many studies have been done to estimate the frequency of

IBD. About 120,000 people in the United States are diagnosed annually with IBD.

The number is most likely higher than that. The majority of cases might not even be recorded, and there is much misdiagnosis.

Both of these diseases appeared in isolated cases several centuries ago, but didn't attract medical interest until the last half of the 19th century. Ulcerative colitis was first described and named in 1875 and Crohn's disease in 1913, but it's only in the last ten to fifteen years that people have begun to talk about them openly as they do with other diseases such as heart disease, diabetes, and even cancer. In the past, not many people felt comfortable talking about diarrhea, bloody bowel movements, or the need for frequent, urgent trips to the bathroom. Because so many people still feel uncomfortable talking about IBD, they probably don't visit the doctor to get diagnosed, but their IBD still exists. It's likely that more people suffer from some form of IBD than most other diseases in the world combined.

## Who Gets IBD?

My doctor says studies suggest only certain people usually get IBD. Is that true?

Yes, that is correct. People who are sick haven't treated their bodies with healthful choices, and IBD can be the result. These people have neither eaten healthfully, nor have they lived a healthy lifestyle. In fact, given the way people eat today, it's very likely nearly everyone eating the common diet will get some form of IBD at some point. There are emotional and mental issues that can be part of the cause, but the main cause of IBD is dietary! This is without a doubt a 100% fact. You cannot catch it from anyone, and you can't have IBD if you're eating a healthy diet, living and thinking a healthy lifestyle.

There are some studies that show how IBD affects different peoples in different parts of the world. It's more prevalent in some parts of the world and more present in certain cultures than in others, but everyone with an unhealthy diet can get it.

There are also studies documenting that there are more cases of IBD in developed countries than in underdeveloped countries. If the people running these studies and the medical community were to understand the connection between diet and IBD, they would realize that eating richer (processed) foods and having the money to overeat are the cause. But instead, they try to justify it by saying poorer people are less likely to seek treatment for disease. That doesn't make sense; people aren't suffering from IBD because they haven't sought medical treatment.

## Can anyone at any age get IBD?

IBD can start at any age, but usually begins in the late teens or early adulthood, or, less often in middle age. At least that's when the disease becomes such a problem for people that they can no longer live with it and go to the doctor. It usually starts at a much younger age. Many people believe all diseases start in the colon, and the first disease everyone will get is some form of IBS or IBD. Given the way people eat today, most people in the civilized world are likely to develop some form of IBS or IBD at some point, unless there are dramatic dietary improvements.

## What about young children? How common is it for them to get diagnosed with IBD?

About 20 percent of adults with IBD exhibited symptoms before age 15. This is changing fast. With the terrible diets kids have today and the misinformation parents have about health, more and more kids are experiencing signs of IBD and IBS; more and more kids are getting diagnosed with IBD. The disease is still rarely diagnosed in children before age 10 unless another family member has it. Most diseases start slowly and build up over the years; and most kids are not tested at such a young age because the signs aren't always as severe as when they grow older, but

34

that doesn't mean they don't have IBD. A major sign is when very young children are not developing at the same rate as other children their age. It is essential for children with IBD to get adequate nutrition so that their growth and development are not stunted.

**Living with IBD or Without It! The Choice Is Yours.**

As I stated earlier, you do not have to live with IBD for the rest of your life. So many books today teach how to live it for the rest of your life, but if you cure it, you don't have to worry about that. However, during the time you're working on your cure, you may have to live with IBD for a short time. Here are some questions that address this issue:

If I suffer from IBD, will it be very hard to deal with people and life? Will my life turn into a hard road?

If you listen to your doctor, this is true, but if you listen to and adopt nature's cure I explain in Part Three of this book, there is no need to worry about anything. A flare-up, or an IBD attack, can be the worst feeling in the world. It makes it very hard to do anything, so the answer is to avoid attacks. In nature's cure, I explain how to do just that — forever!

If I have IBD, does that mean I will be sick all the time?

No, you will be well between attacks. For any given patient, attacks, or flare-ups, may occur frequently (every few weeks) or rarely (every few years). A person may have multiple flare-ups one year and then none for several years, or any other irregular pattern you can imagine. The average risk of a flare-up is about 10% per year for UC and 30% for Crohn's. I have recently met someone who said he didn't have a flare-up for ten years, then, all of a sudden, he had one. But he wasn't eating a healthy diet. I've never met anyone who has done what I suggested who didn't get better. There are always exceptions, and everyone should ultimately be treated individually, but nature's cure for IBD will bring an improvement to all who learn it and adopt it.

## How bad can the urge to go to the bathroom get?

Let me start by saying, I understand because I've been there. It's very hard to talk about because it has to deal with the bathroom and diarrhea, blood and mucus, but it's important to understand that you're not alone. A bathroom will quickly become your best friend and the most needed thing in your life. The urge will be so strong, you might feel you will not be able to make it, even worse, you might not make it. Rubbing my belly used to help sometimes, or trying to redirect my feelings as long as I could until I was able to get to a bathroom also helped; but, in most cases, the urge will just come upon you quickly. Usually, the longer a person is in an attack, the worse the urges will become. But the more you learn how to control them, the more prepared you'll be. At first you might have control over the urges, but if you don't take care of the problem, the urges will take control over you.

## Sometimes a bathroom is not within reach; what do I do then?

Hopefully, you will quickly follow my suggestions in Part Three, but if you don't, or if you do, and you're not totally healed yet, once you have an uncontrollable urge, pray that there is a bathroom nearby. Otherwise, it can get ugly. I understand this so well because I've experienced IBD attacks without being near a bathroom, and it can be a really unpleasant experience. I spent most of my time complaining and saying, "Why me?" until I decided to take control of my health. Now, I no longer have any problems with IBD. Although I have faith in what I'm doing, those attacks were so scary that I still pray everyday that I'll never have to go though them again.

## Do you have any suggestions for help when in this situation?

If I recall correctly, if you get a note from your doctor, you can get a handicap sticker and park in handicap spots. That would be of great help in certain situations. Try to plan your day well so you have a bathroom near you throughout the day. Unfortunately, some businesses just don't get it, they don't understand and will not let the public use the bathroom in their shops. Carrying a small note to show them might help so they do understand.

## What about the blood loss in my stool? Can that cause an iron deficiency, or make me anemic?

Whenever there is blood in the stool, there can be a loss of iron. This can lead to anemia, which means there is a reduced number of red blood cells. Red blood cells carry oxygen throughout the blood. When more iron is lost than is taken in, there can be a loss of up to an ounce and a half (40 milliliters) of blood a day in the stool without it being seen. If the bleeding comes from high enough up in the GI tract, the blood is thoroughly mixed in with the stool. Losing a small amount of blood on a daily basis can lead to iron-deficiency anemia over a period of several months.

No one with a recent onset of UC should have an iron deficiency that causes anemia, and people with Crohn's disease very rarely become anemic. Even though blood is obviously in the stool, the amount is almost always less than you think; it takes very little bright red fluid to color the toilet bowl water red! Unless bleeding is truly heavy, the bone marrow is able to use available stores of iron to keep the red blood cell count in the normal range.

If the bleeding is heavy, this can be a big problem. Other than doctors prescribing drugs and supplements, you have only one other choice — to prevent the blood from getting into the stool. The best way to do that would be to follow the suggestions for a natural cure in Part Three. This will take care of any and all nutrient problems.

## It must be so hard for a young child to deal with such pain.

Children, particularly teenagers, are very anxious not to be seen as different from their peers; their self-consciousness and intolerance of other children often lead to a degree of isolation. People of all ages who suffer from IBD can tend to isolate themselves, but it's very common for kids and teenagers with this illness to do so. We must make sure the kids understand there is a cure, and the way it's going to be accomplished be explained to them. We must help them to heal.

## Is there really a cure for IBD?

**The cause of IBD is unknown, and there is no known cure for anyone who has it, according to my medical doctor.**

That is correct; medical doctors do not know the cause of IBD, but I have learned it the hard way — by getting it and getting rid of it. Since doctors don't know the cause, how could they know the cure? I know both how to avoid it, and how to cure it if you've already been diagnosed with it. I've been in remission for years, as have many people who have learned what I have and are doing what I'm doing.

I will talk more about prevention and the cure in Part Three, but right now I'd like to talk about the cause.

IBD, as most other diseases, is diet related. There are only a few types of food that are truly natural to the human body. When I say natural, I mean foods our bodies can easily use without having to overwork. When we eat unnatural foods, our bodies have to work very hard to digest them which creates a great deal of stress. Here's the way it works:

## Stress vs. Vitality

When the body is healthy, it has a lot of vitality and energy. When the body is overstressed, it loses vitality, and all that stress equals a major discomfort. Another word for discomfort in the body is disease. Everyone has genetic weakness in his/her chemical makeup, and it's usually the weakest part of the body that suffers the most, or first, when we do things that are unnatural. It's like playing Russian roulette — the bullet is in the gun, but unless you pull the trigger, it can never hurt you. It works the same way with genetic weaknesses: as long as we don't pull the trigger, the weakness can never hurt us. Once we pull the trigger, we will suffer a great discomfort — a disease. The trigger is stress. The more stress we have, the more discomfort we'll have, and the worse the disease will be. In my final cure for IBD in Part Three, I will explain what that trigger is, how to avoid it, and how to cure yourself if you have disease. I know it's tempting, but please don't go to Part Three until you've finished reading all of the questions and answers here in Part Two. This will help to give you a better understanding of the final cure. I'm so sure this cure will work, but it also depends on how completely the patient understands it. It has worked for me and many others. Doctors do not know what it is because they are often close-minded. You can relieve yourself of all worry because there is a natural cure for IBD, and you're just a few pages away from learning and applying it.

## I have a bowel movement once a day, so I'm not constipated.

Just because you have a bowel movement once a day doesn't mean you're not constipated. If you eat six times a day and have one bowel movement a day, that is a serious form of constipation. There are many early warning signs of getting some form of IBS or IBD; constipation is one of the most obvious. When a person has IBD, there is a good chance the number of trips to the bathroom are going to be many, but before the attacks start, if the person is constipated, that is not good either. Everybody should ideally have a bowel movement at least two to three times a day, depending on how much he/she is eating.

### ...AND THE TRUTH SHALL SET YOU FREE

## But my doctor says there is no known medical cure for IBD.

That is also correct. How can doctors have a cure for something when they don't know its cause? I know the cause, and I've been privileged to learn the natural cure.

## According to medical studies and my doctors, the only thing a person with IBD can do to control this disease is to take drugs.

That is true. Doctors are in the business of controlling diseases of all types, and they do so with drugs. The problem is the drugs are harmful and have side effects. Even if the drugs control the disease, they do not cure the patient. Just as doctors are in the business of controlling disease, I'm in the business of teaching its natural cure.

## My doctor says, if the drugs don't work, I'll have to get surgery to remove the infected part of my colon.

That's just like doctors. If they can't control it, they say, "Get rid of it." We need all of our body parts to be as healthy and to stay as healthy as possible. Years ago, surgery used to be a last resort, but now many doctors are using it commonly as a first resort when it comes to IBD and many other diseases. There are many reasons for this, but rest assured, surgery is not needed in most cases of IBD. With the natural IBD cure, you will be 100% well without surgery, or the need to take drugs ever again. Doctors even go so far as to say, "Sometimes surgery is the ONLY choice."

CRAZY! It's just the only one they've learned in medical school. Doctors are very willing to remove your colon, rectum, and if that happens, the anus must also be removed. You choose: would you rather try a natural cure, or take the doctor's drugs, or have a doctor take out your colon? I am sure nature's cure is the best of these choices, and it's the only one that works. Just to let you know what doctors do to remove the colon or parts of it: they make incisions in the abdomen and the perineum, the area between the anus and the genitals.

Sometimes doctors will call patients lucky if they don't need a complete removal of the colon and rectum. If the rectum can remain (known as a subtotal colectomy), then the doctor will say it wasn't bad. If the whole colon and rectum come out, it is known as a total colectomy. And, sometimes, a subtotal removal can mean the entire colon and most of the rectum come out.

Most doctors will only suggest surgery if medical therapy has failed to control the disease adequately, or if cancer has been found. But many of them jump the gun and cut too soon. It's different with UC and Crohn's. Surgery in the case of UC would completely get rid of the disease, but since Crohn's disease can occur in other parts of the body, surgery will not assure a patient of a 100% recovery. Surgery for UC involves removing most, or all, of the colon. Surgery for Crohn's disease depends on where in the GI tract the disease occurs.

## My doctor says, a person with IBD is at a higher risk of developing colon cancer.

That may be true. If patients keep up the lifestyle they're used to and continue to build on the stress level, there will be two choices left: get the colon taken out, or develop colon cancer.

## DIET AND IBD

In this section I expose the lack of nutritional understanding many medical doctors have. It may seem as if I'm bashing doctors here, but I'm not doing anything but telling the truth. Some doctors are great at what they do and are very needed: emergency room doctors, cases of spinal cord injury, etc. But if I create an illness in my body by eating an unhealthy diet, what is going to cure it is to stop eating unhealthy foods and replace them with healthy foods, not a doctor's ideas of how to control my illness.

## Is there a connection between diet and IBD?

Yes, there is a big connection. In fact, that is the most important connection. IBD is a disease that is caused mostly by a stressful diet. The cure is also related to diet. In the next chapter, the connection between diet and IBD is explained.

## My doctor says that diet has no role is causing or curing IBD.

Your doctor is wrong, and that is a statement I will stand behind 100%. If your doctor tells you this, I suggest you get a new doctor fast. I hope you understand, after having read up to this point that there is a big connection between diet and IBD, and most doctors don't know much about either one. The problem is that students in medical schools receive too little instruction in nutrition and don't learn about healing by nutritional means.

## If I have IBD, is it true that I can suffer from a malabsorption of vitamins and minerals?

It is possible to suffer from malabsorption if you listen to a doctor's advice, it is also possible if you listen to my advice, but it is highly unlikely that you will suffer from any malabsorpition at all after following my suggestions. Nature's cure for IBD is designed to give the body every nutrient it needs for healing, and at the same time any possible lack of important nutrients is avoided.

Malabsorption is very common when inflammation affects

the colon because inflammation usually gets in the way of nutrient absorption.

The inflammation also can cause diarrhea that can cause a loss of the body's electrolytes and mineral salts needed to maintain correct fluid balance, nervous system functions and general health.

Malabsorption can affect people in many different ways, depending on the nutrient in which they are deficient. In children with IBD, it can affect growth and development since they usually don't eat enough, and the nutrients in their food aren't being absorbed. In adults, since they're already grown, it will show up as laziness, or an inability to maintain weight. Sometimes women with IBD don't maintain enough body fat and stop menstruation — a problem that can also arise from a lack of protein.

Long term consequences of malabsorption can include vitamin and mineral deficiencies, but nature's cure is the optimum way to avoid any problems and to be assured of getting the highest quality nutrients. Deficiencies accrue from the doctors' approach to handling IBD. The deficiencies from a malabsorption problem start slowly, but in time become worse. Usually, deficiencies manifest as rather vague symptoms we all experience once in a while. Irritability and depression come first, but the other most common symptoms are cracking of the lips at the corners of the mouth, dull hair, weak or brittle fingernails, chills or feeling cold easily, a lack of energy and recurring headaches. We all feel these symptoms from time to time, but if you have IBD and any of these symptoms persist for days, see your doctor for a diagnosis, and then seek a nutritional counselor.

## My doctor says I need to take vitamin and mineral supplements.

Your doctor is partly correct. There are certain whole live food supplements that I, too, suggest can be helpful, but they are different from those doctors would recommend. I would suggest enzymes, probiotics and mineral supplements. Your doctor would most likely recommend vitamin supplements. If you're eating a diet that consists of a good variety of high quality foods, you should be getting all the vitamins your body needs. In Part Three, I talk about the supplements that would be helpful.

## Dehydration

Your body can either be hydrated or dehydrated; make sure to drink enough water every day. People with IBD tend to be even more dehydrated than average people who are usually dehydrated anyway. This is because when IBD sufferers have many bowel movements with a lot of diarrhea, their bodies tend to lose more water than average. I would suggest keeping well hydrated by drinking a good amount of water throughout the day. It is not suggested that you drink with your meals; drink an hour before or an hour afterwards. An hour should be the time allowed between your meals and your drinking. When you drink any liquid with your meals, you're diluting your saliva. That's where digestion starts, and when you dilute your saliva you're stressing your body to work harder than necessary.

## Medication and Nutrition

Taking medications usually increases one or more nutritional requirements; no medication has yet been developed that decreases nutritional requirements. Medications used for IBD range from corticosteroids to many other prescription drugs. They are all only quick answers, but, in the long run, many of them cause deficiencies by removing too many nutrients from the body. This is another reason why many doctors will prescribe some vitamin supplements — not that they know about nutrition, but because they know the medication they're prescribing will cause vitamin and mineral losses.

**After an IBD attack, I lose a lot of weight. To put on weight, my doctor says I have to eat more food, more protein and fats.**

This is what I'm talking about when I say doctors know very little about the connection between diet and health. Doctors might be concerned with weight issues, and if you want to put on weight, then stuffing your body with high fat foods will, of course, add weight. But instead, I think we should focus on muscle weight rather than fat weight. You must exercise, rest, have good nutrition, but most of all, you must cleanse and heal before the healthy weight can come back. Eat mostly green vegetables. When you are in an IBD flare-up, I suggest eating these foods in blended form so the fiber will not bother you. A blended salad or green drink is excellent. There is more information about this in Part Three. Once you follow my suggestions, you might lose some weight when starting, but in the long run, you will be healthy, cured of IBD, and your weight will balance out.

**My doctor told me it's harmful to eat foods such as fruits and vegetables raw.**

Your doctor is uninformed in this area. Take my diet for example: it consists entirely of raw fruits and vegetables. There are some harmful raw foods you can eat, but raw fresh organically grown fruits and vegetables are the best for you, as long as they taste good. Chances are that if you get low quality foods, neither ripe nor fresh, they won't taste good. But getting high quality fresh, ripe organic raw foods will not only taste great, but will also be great for you. During an IBD flare-up, the fiber of fruits and vegetables might bother some people, but in blended or juiced form, there is no healthier food for you.

45

My doctor said eating raw foods, especially nuts and seeds, is bad for me, even dangerous. He is a doctor, shouldn't he know all about diet?

Why should he? Most doctors know very little about a natural diet. If you follow the doctor's dietary guidelines, there's a good chance you will end up very sick. If you listen to my suggestions for a natural diet, there is a very good chance you will get better. Just as with whole vegetables and fruits, if during a flare-up, nuts and seeds are eaten in their whole form, they might further stress your condition. But in blended form, such as in nut milks and nut butters, nuts and seeds are fine and very health promoting for IBD sufferers.

Won't I suffer from a deficiency if I eat only a vegetarian diet?

No you won't. Everything your body needs is found in a vegetarian diet, as long as it includes a good variety of fresh fruits and vegetables. Raw fruits, vegetables, nuts and seeds contain everything your body needs. I've been eating this way for years and just took a blood test. The test results show that I have no deficiencies at all.

What about TPN (Total Parenteral Nutrition)?

Doctors, when they have no idea what to do, give their patients TPN, which stands for Total Parenteral Nutrition. This diet is given by a route other than the GI tract. It is reserved mainly for patients who are acutely ill, such as those with severe IBD, but in my view, doctors who have no idea at all about nutrition administer it. There may be some instances where TPN might help, but it's not necessary. A raw diet, as described in nature's cure for IBD, will keep the patient well nourished.

## What about lactose intolerance and allergies to dairy products and other foods?

The body is allergic to all foods that are not fit for human consumption, but also has an amazing power to adapt. Just because we can digest a food without having a reaction doesn't mean we're not allergic to it. If you have IBD, you are definitely eating foods you're allergic to, and once you stop eating those foods, you'll find you're feeling better. Remember, health doesn't start with what you add to your diet, it's what you leave out that counts. Find out which foods are bad for IBD, eliminate them from your diet, and you should find yourself healed in no time. Most often, dairy products and products containing wheat are the most common foods that cause IBD, or make it worse. I would start by avoiding these foods and watching the great results.

## OTHER FACTORS

## My doctor says there is no evidence that stress of any kind can cause an IBD attack.

There is substantial evidence that stress to the body, physically, mentally, emotionally and spiritually, can cause an IBD attack. Stress is one of the prime causes of IBD. Stress and discomfort arc other ways of saying dis-ease. No matter how well people eat, if the stress in their lives is not reduced, they will still be at risk to experience the pain and suffering of IBD.

## What about emotions and IBD?

A person with IBD can become emotionally drained. The entire digestive system is intricately involved with emotions. People can get sick on a ride, or seeing a movie with lots of graphic gore. Visual signals to the brain can trigger a major reaction in the stomach and digestive system. Since the bowels respond to emotions, it follows that emotional upset, or stress, can make inflamed bowels worse.

## Okay, what about other factors?

## Other than the food I eat, or the stress I cause, is there anything else that can be a factor?

There are many minor factors that are different for all of us. That's what makes us who we are. The key is, before focusing on those minor issues, you should concentrate on the major issues outlined in this book.

One major issue I haven't focused on in this book, but I'm in the process of working on for a future book, is the emotional/spiritual connection to disease. The instructions for living a healthy life, on everything from how we eat, to how we think, to how we act, are all found in the greatest health book ever written: The Bible. When we live a life that goes against the teachings of The Bible, it will affect our health on one level or another. Just as important as physical food, is spiritual food, and the best spiritual food can be gotten from developing a personal relationship with God. I found the best way to do this is to read God's commandments; live them and pray everyday.

## Can heredity be a factor?

Some people believe that genes may predispose a person to IBD, and that genetics do play a role. Anything is possible, but as I've stated time and time again, IBD is a dietary illness. We all have genetic weaknesses, and if we pull the trigger they will get us, but if we never pull the trigger, they won't. The trigger in this case is the same trigger that's been around for so long: eating unhealthy food.

## OTHER ISSUES INVOLVED IN LIVING WITH IBD

### If I have IBD, can I still be fit and active?

Of course you can. Obviously, when you're in the midst of a flare-up, you wouldn't be able or even want to be involved in many activities. But if you don't get any flare-ups, or only very few, there is no reason you wouldn't be able to be fit and active, as long as you are eating well and making sure to get enough rest.

### What is the outlook for IBD patients?

From the point of view of being able to learn and adopt a natural lifestyle, the outlook has never been better. More and more people are improving the way they eat and are on their way toward a more healthful lifestyle. Eating according to my suggestions for a natural diet, even to some degree, works wonders. However, there is no known medical cure for IBD.

*Most people today learn "health care" through mass media instead of listening to their own inner feelings. Become aware of your body's innate capacity for healing, and break the cycle of this mad society.*

### I've read some books about IBD written by medical doctors. In their books, they say things you have found to be bad advice. You call the medical position "crazy." But they are doctors, and this is serious. What medical background do you have? Why do you think your information is better than theirs?

Many people are scared to stop listening to doctors. That means they would have to take responsibility for their own health, and they couldn't blame someone when something goes wrong. If you're listening to a doctor, chances are something will go wrong. I know advice based on the doctors' information is not good because the results of following it are not good. That's the bottom line; and we all need good results. My advice, based on an understanding of nature, is very different from that of medical doctors, and the results are very different also. There is no medical cure for IBD, yet I have cured myself of it, as have many others, after having discovered a natural healing path. Good results count!

Many people today have such closed minds and only listen to what doctors say. Well, most of what doctors say, and the things many of them suggest, are very scary, to say the least. If I were to tell someone to do something, I would be questioned because I don't wear a white coat or have a medical degree. But I do have a degree in results. Not too many doctors can say that. What are results? Doctors also get results, but the results they get create a challenge to the body. Doctors want to control disease with drugs; they accomplish that and call it results. I don't look at controlling a disease as really long lasting results; results to me are curing a disease, and those are the results that I've gotten through a correct understanding of nature.

It's very scary that people put so much trust in doctors when IBD is a dietary illness. Unfortunately, most American doctors don't study the connection between diet and illness. Just a few examples of this: I recently read a book about IBD written by a medical doctor, and I still can't believe my eyes as to what he wrote, but this is no joke. Here's an excerpt:

*"People with IBD often discover that they feel better if they don't eat. Unfortunately, this worsens the weight loss many patients experience. Some patients mistakenly believe that spicy or greasy food should be avoided, but then their diet becomes boring. This can lead to eating even less food and losing more weight."*

This doctor actually justifies eating spicy and greasy food. If he had any idea about the connection between diet and IBD, he would know that greasy and spicy foods are some of the worst foods, not only for a person with IBD, but for anyone.

In the same book, the doctor spoke about how some people experience relief from symptoms when they go on a liquid diet for a short time. I agree with this. I feel a liquid diet of fresh vegetable juices and blended salads are excellent, but that is not what this doctor was talking about. As I kept reading, I again couldn't believe my eyes when I read the liquid diet the doctor was suggesting. For a clear fluid diet, he suggests jelly, tea with sugar, chicken broth, and beef broth; for a full fluid diet: strained oatmeal with milk and sugar, coffee with sugar and cream, creamed soup and ice cream.

This is some of the worst advice for anyone with IBD, but, then, to make matters worse, the doctor goes on to say that once the patient stops the liquid diet and goes back to eating a regular diet, it should consist of animal products, milk and candy. It's no wonder that someone who eats this way will become sick and deficient in nutrients.

Doctors who put people on this type of diet, as they usually do, will also suggest a meal replacement shake or drink as a supplement. The answer to getting what we're missing in our diet is not in a supplement drink. Eating a high quality diet is the answer.

Not only do doctors suggest a diet of very low quality food, but then they suggest low quality nutritional products and drinks filled with dairy, sugar, corn syrup, fat from corn oil, and other harmful products. What doctors are telling people to do is just crazy.

Now, I know what you're most likely thinking: that it's just this one doctor who wrote a certain book that is giving bad advice, and not all medical doctors are that bad. YES THEY ARE! When it comes to nutrition and IBD, most medical doctors will suggest the same things that I've quoted above.

## Of all the crazy things you've heard, what was the craziest treatment for IBD?

I've read some pretty bad nutritional advise about how to handle IBD, but the worst I've read comes from another book, written, by another medical doctor. The doctor was addressing the topic of weight loss and IBD patients. The doctor wrote that there is no reason for IBD patients to avoid spicy foods because many people with IBD are underweight, particularly when they have been ill, and fat is an excellent source of energy. So the doctor said that to keep weight on the patients, they should eat extra amounts of fatty foods.

The doctor says that people who are underweight can't afford to cut back on the number of calories they eat, so they should eat even if they don't have an appetite — that it's okay. He even suggested the patient with IBD eat fried foods because they taste better, so the person will eat more, and that spices also need to be added to make the food more appealing. According to this doctor, spices improve taste, which helps to increase food intake and eating fried foods will help the person compensate for the weight loss.

The doctor, in a confusing statement, writes that he doesn't suggest eating a high fat diet because it may increase the risk of heart disease, but in trying to regain weight, it is generally harmless to eat an increased amount of fat.

Then to top it off, he says when he has a patient who is having trouble gaining weight after an IBD flare-up, he often suggests high fat, high energy foods such as bacon and eggs, potato chips and various fried foods.

If anyone with some natural nutritional knowledge were to think about what this doctor is saying, this advice would be found very dangerous, even crazy, and certainly confusing.

## If you have all the answers and the cure for IBD and are so sure of them, why won't medical doctors listen to you?

For one, they won't listen to me because I don't have the schooling to be a doctor. I'm just an average guy, and what doctor is going to listen to a person who didn't go to school to learn to be a doctor? Some doctors have the best intentions and want to find the right answers. There are a good number of doctors out there who have found nature's cure and apply it. Many doctors are looking for what is best for the patient, but they just haven't been exposed to the overwhelming information supporting successful natural healing. I'm sure if they had been, most of them wouldn't argue with nature's cure and would incorporate it into their practice. Unfortunately, there are many doctors who have different motives. Remember: doctors get paid a lot of money when people are sick. The sicker people are, the more money they make. Doctors in the United States do not get paid to keep people healthy. The status quo of sickness is better for their pocketbooks because if they knew how to keep people healthy, who would make appointments to see them?

## When will the medical community wake to the truth about IBD and all diseases?

Unless they can find a way to make money through keeping people healthy, don't expect the way doctors treat their patients to change anytime soon. The way it is now, doctors would lose a lot of money if people were to eat more healthfully and consequently grew healthier. Once again, this is not the agenda of all doctors, and many doctors justify their practice by the money they get paid. They are well worth it. But for most doctors, this is not the case. If it were, they wouldn't be looking for so many answers, they would have them and be using them.

**People need to know they have a choice.  Spread the truth. Spread the cure!**

The information you now have is not the end;  it's just the beginning.  It all depends on what you do with it.

When I first found out I had IBD,  I had no idea what it was; I just knew it was the most hurtful thing in the world.  I was blessed to find the correct information to help me cure myself and keep healthy.  If it weren't for those special people out there who had spread the information I needed,  I never would have found it.  The more correct information people have about how nature works,  the better off they will be.  If medical doctors are the only ones telling us what is right and wrong,  how can we ever learn anything about regaining our natural state of health? Now that you have this information,  once you cure yourself, and you will when you follow the guidelines in this book,  don't stop there.  Get this information out to as many people as you can, and help them heal just as you have.

# Part Three

## Nature's Cure for IBD, and Why It Works

I believe no two people are in the same place at the same time, so there will not always be the same exact answer for everyone. I have found the suggestions below to help improve, and many times completely heal IBD symptoms. If you try these suggestions and don't have results, don't give up. There is an answer. There is a natural way to overcome IBD. Have patience, stay strong, and keep searching untill you achieve total health. Don't accept anything but the best. Do the best you can, and leave the rest up to God.

### DIET

The food you choose to put in your body is a big part of the healing process. Even more important than the food you put in is the food you leave out of your dict. Below arc my top suggestions for a successful natural IBD cure:

### Tip #1

**Eliminate all dairy products from your diet.**

Health does not begin with what you add to your life, or your diet; it's what you leave out that counts even more. That's where the real healing begins. Leave out the things that are causing your illness in the first place, and you'll be much better off. Of all foods, dairy products are probably the most harmful for the IBD sufferer. Milk, cheese, ice cream and even yogurt should all be avoided. Isn't it odd that these same products are harmful for everyone, not just people with IBD? Some people think they shouldn't drink milk because they're allergic to it. I have news for you, every human being on this planet is allergic to animal milk, and they will all get sick from it sooner or later. Neither does it help that the people who process the milk put deadly additives into each container.

## Tip #2

**Eliminate all wheat products.**

Throughout my whole life, I was told that wheat was good for me. When I found out it's not only bad for me, but most likely a cause of IBD, I couldn't believe it. Soon after I began to avoid wheat products, I got 100% better. When I wanted to find out what the problem was with wheat, I read a book titled *Against the Grain*, and it really shed some light on the situation. The book talks about Ciliac disease — an allergy to wheat gluten. Great book. It wasn't easy to stop eating wheat, but it's the last thing I ate before I officially changed my diet to all healthy eating. Now I know I'm fine; as long as I don't eat wheat or dairy, I'm healthy.

## Tip #3

**Eliminate all flour products.**

This is hard because the common world tells us we should be eating wheat, but now I've just let you know how bad wheat is for someone with IBD. Your first thought is probably to put down this book and get some white bread because Paul said wheat was no good. Well, in a different way, all flour products: bread, pasta, and cereal are unhealthy for you. Even if they don't contain wheat, it's still wise to avoid flour products.

## Tip #4

**Reduce the amount of sugar you eat, and only eat high quality sugar such as found in fruits. NO processed sugar.**

Processed sugar is another thing you should get out of your diet. Instead, replace the processed sugar with the good quality sugar found in fruits. But be careful. I've found that even when eating the best foods for the body, if you overeat, it's not going to be healthful. Stick to natural, unprocessed food, and you will be fine.

## Tip #5

**Reduce the amount of bad fat in your diet, and stop eating cooked or animal fats.**

There is good fat, and there is bad fat. The health promoting fats are in plant foods and should be eaten raw. The unhealthy ones are any cooked fats and animal fats. Once you realize this, it's easy to make wise decisions about the type of fats to eat and which ones to avoid. Beware, there are many bad fats hiding in packaged foods today.

## Tip #6

**Use the principles of food combining for all your meals.**

Your food choices are always very important, but to improve your health, you can keep things as easy as possible for your body. The more you make your organs work to digest food, the more stress you will add. The less work your organs have to do to process the food, the better. Eating foods in an order that will keep it easy on the body is very helpful. That's what food combining is. There are many different types of raw foods, and different types will take different lengths of time to digest. Your body will have to work harder to digest foods if you eat them in poor combinations. You want your body to waste as little energy as possible. For this reason, it's important to combine your food properly. There are many books written about food combining. I suggest you read some of them to learn as much as you can about the subject. To help you understand appropriate food combinations and to make it simpler, always remember to eat liquid foods with other liquid foods, and more dense foods with other dense foods.

The best foods for the human body are ripe, organic fruits and vegetables. The best fruits and vegetables for the human body will contain the highest water content possible. A good way to measure water content is to put any food through a juicer. The more liquid that comes out, the higher the water content of that food and the more beneficial that food is for you. Picture your body as a juicer. If eaten in its raw state, there will be no better choice for the human body than high water content foods.

Cooking will evaporate most of the water and make even the most perfect food dense, dull, and dead. That's only part of what makes it so bad. Try putting a piece of bread into a juicer, and you'll see the juicer working very hard, but still nothing will come out. If you continue, eventually the juicer will break, just as your body will get diseased if you continue to eat cooked foods.

When you eat one food as your entire meal (a mono-diet), you don't have to think about food combining. However, if you're going to eat many different kinds of food in the same meal, you should study and follow the rules of food-combining. The following chart will inform you about food-combining.

(Chart complements of Dave Klien)

# Food Combining Chart

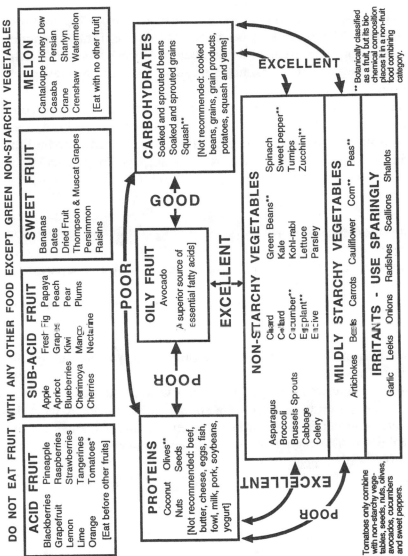

**DO NOT EAT FRUIT WITH ANY OTHER FOOD EXCEPT GREEN NON-STARCHY VEGETABLES**

**ACID FRUIT**
Blackberries    Pineapple
Grapefruit      Raspberries
Lemon           Strawberries
Lime            Tangerines
Orange          Tomatoes*
[Eat before other fruits]

**SUB-ACID FRUIT**
Apple       Fresh Fig   Papaya
Apricot     Grapes      Peach
Blueberries Kiwi        Pear
Cherimoya   Mango       Plums
Cherries    Nectarine

**SWEET FRUIT**
Bananas
Dates
Dried Fruit
Thompson & Muscat Grapes
Persimmon
Raisins

**MELON**
Cantaloupe  Honey Dew
Casaba      Persian
Crane       Sharlyn
Crenshaw    Watermelon

[Eat with no other fruit]

**CARBOHYDRATES**
Soaked and sprouted beans
Soaked and sprouted grains
Squash**

[Not recommended: cooked beans, grains, grain products, potatoes, squash and yams]

**OILY FRUIT**
Avocado
A superior source of essential fatty acids]

**PROTEINS**
Coconut   Olives**
Nuts      Seeds

[Not recommended: beef, butter, cheese, eggs, fish, fowl, milk, pork, soybeans, yogurt]

**NON-STARCHY VEGETABLES**
Asparagus          Chard     Green Beans**   Spinach
Broccoli           Collard   Kale            Sweet pepper**
Brussels Sprouts   Cucumber**Kohl-rabi       Turnips
Cabbage            Eggplant**Lettuce         Zucchini**
Celery             Endive    Parsley

**MILDLY STARCHY VEGETABLES**
Artichokes   Beets   Carrots   Cauliflower   Corn**   Peas**

**IRRITANTS - USE SPARINGLY**
Garlic   Leeks   Onions   Radishes   Scallions   Shallots

EXCELLENT
GOOD
POOR
POOR
POOR
EXCELLENT
EXCELLENT
POOR

** Botanically classified as a fruit, but its biochemical composition places it in a non-fruit food combining category.

* Tomatoes only combine with non-starchy vegetables, seeds, nuts, olives, avocados, cucumbers and sweet peppers.

## Tip #7

**Nut milks**

Make a blended almond drink. When healing from IBD with this blended almond drink, it is important that the drink be strained and smooth. If you can find raw peeled almonds that would help, but be careful. Most blanched almonds in the store say raw when in fact they are pre-boiled. If you are not 100% sure the almonds are raw, you may use unpeeled almonds. Either way, peeled or unpeeled, soak them for up to 8 hours before using them. Also, do your best to use organic almonds if you can. You can find the recipe for this nut milk under recipes on page 75.

## Tip #8

**Blended foods (purees)**

Blending is the easiest and most efficient way to prepare food that is both nourishing and easy to digest.

Liquids are not always what we think they are. A blend of bananas and apple juice does not make banana-apple juice. It makes a puree of bananas. Just because solids are reduced into liquid form doesn't mean they disappear. Yes, you are eating solid food, only in tiny pieces. After all, where does the banana fiber go? That illustrates the difference between blending and juicing. A blender purees or liquefies a solid food. A juicer extracts the water content from the fruit or vegetable and separates it from the pulp. The higher the solid (fiber) content of a liquid, the harder it is to digest.

## Tip #9

**Eat less, not more.**

The studies are out; the proof is in. The less we eat, the better off we are. But the trick is, the food we are eating must be of good quality. If we are eating good quality food, we only need small amounts because everything we need is right in there. But, when we eat low quality foods, we are not giving the body what it needs, and we will overeat. Eating fresh ripe raw fruits, vegetables, nuts, and seeds, raw and as close to nature as possible will assure that you are giving your body the highest quality foods.

*"In general, mankind, since the improvement of cookery, eats twice as much as nature requires"*
*- Benjamin Franklin*

The big problem is overeating. The body takes what it needs and has to work hard to get rid of the rest. Most of the time so much is eaten in excess that the body cannot keep up with eliminating all the waste.

How much are people eating? And if the waste doesn't come out of the body where is it going? It putrefies and ferments.

**The Digestive and Elimination Tract**

The digestive and elimination tract is one long tube from your mouth to your anus, just shy of 30 feet long. There is only one way in and one way out. This tube is often referred to as the alimentary canal or tract, which includes the mouth, esophagus, stomach, duodenum, small intestine, large intestine, rectum and anus.

Average Americans suffer from at least one type of disease/discomfort to some part of their digestive tract. The result is most often either a polyp, diverticulitis, bleeding fissures, IBD and even colon cancer. Up to 50% of Americans have polyps in their colons. A polyp is a tumor that arises from the bowel surface and protrudes into the inside of the colon. Polyps can eventually transform into malignant cancerous tumors.

People are just eating way too much food, and it isn't getting any better. People are eating more and more when they should be eating less. A recent study confirms that the average American eats way too much food. In a lifetime, the average American consumes:

12 three thousand pound cows

6 whole pigs

3,000 chickens, turkeys and other birds

3,000 fish, sea creatures and sea scavengers

30,000 quarts of cow's milk

30,000 aspirin/pain killers

20,000 over the counter and prescription drugs

2,000 gallons of alcohol

In one year he/she might well consume:

hundreds of pounds of junk foods consisting of cake, candy, doughnuts and soft drinks. A few hundred pounds of white, refined sugar would be a low estimate.

With all this going in, and not as much coming out because so many people suffer from constipation, much waste sits in the digestive tract. Dead, decaying flesh, junk food and drugs, all of it passing through your digestive tract into your bloodstream, brain, heart, and then out through your liver, bowel and kidneys. Dr. Richard Shultz estimates that this fiber free feast causes average Americans to be seventy thousand bowel movements short in their lifetime. Some doctors would suggest that number to be even higher.

According to Dr. Shultz, colon cancer kills 400% more people than AIDS! It actually kills more men and women in the United States than breast or prostate cancer. Colon-rectal cancer will kill about 60,000 Americans this year with over 150,000 new cases diagnosed. Many people don't like to talk about colon disease or health.

It's going in, but it's not coming out. When we are constipated, the things we put into our bodies will putrefy or ferment causing deadly gases that will back up into the bloodstream causing many problems.

Here is a statement from an excellent book by Dr. Carrington titled *Fasting for Health and Long Life*:

*"When food is not properly digested, it causes trouble! An excess of protein results in putrefaction, an excess of carbohydrates, in fermentation. Both are bad; both result in unpleasant and ultimately serious symptoms. Gases and poisons are formed within the body, which pass into the bloodstream and affect the tissues and organs, and even the delicate nerve cells of the brain. The mental and emotional life are affected, no less than the grosser physical elements. Waste material accumulates, toxins are formed, which poison and block the tiny blood vessels. The body becomes choked with the excess. Desperately, nature tries to get rid of this load by driving the eliminating organs to greater and greater efforts, until they break down under the strain. When this occurs, the patient is already in the throes of illness. He is now a really sick man."*

The average American stores from six to ten pounds of fecal waste in his/her colon, which is not healthy. Constipation is one of the first signs that disease will be happening. In my opinion, overeating which leads to constipation is the beginning of the end. It is the primary cause of nearly every disturbance of the human system. Eat less food, less often, and make sure it's of high quality.

## WHOLE, LIVE FOOD SUPPLEMENTS

Even though I call them supplements, they're not really supplements. They're live foods in supplement form. If you have IBD, even if you're eating a health promoting diet, I highly recommend taking these supplements to ensure your health and healing.

## Tip #1

### Enzymes

To conserve enzymes, eat most of your food raw. Enzymes are protein compounds we need in order to survive. They are involved in nearly every activity that takes place within our bodies, including digestion. Unfortunately, many scientists fail to realize just how necessary enzymes are to human life, and as a result, the importance of including enzymes in the diet is often overlooked.

Enzymes are fragile substances. Cooking food at temperatures higher than 118 degrees destroys its natural enzymes as well as many vitamins needed for optimum health.

Enzymes are divided into two main groups: metabolic and digestive. Metabolic enzymes act as catalysts, promoting or speeding up the numerous chemical reactions in the body. They are also responsible for the building and repairing of cells, among other functions. Digestive enzymes are present in the digestive tract, and are responsible for breaking down food.

Humans are born with a certain number of enzymes; we can also get them from food. Enzymes obtained from raw food help to digest everything we eat. If we don't obtain enough enzymes from our food, we must draw on our supply of metabolic enzymes to aid digestion. This means there are fewer enzymes available for other functions in the body, such as cleansing and repair. This enzyme imbalance eventually leads to illnesses, including allergies, obesity, heart disease and some forms of cancer.

Enzymes are the active ingredients that cure dis-ease. They are the central core of the immune system and necessary for the maintenance of health. It is the enzymatic activity that makes the brain function, the memory work, and keeps the body alive. Adding enzymes supplements to the high quality food you are now eating will assure you are healing optimally.

## Tip #2

### Green super food powders

Many people are not getting enough minerals in their diets. Green vegetables are the best source of minerals. Most people are not eating enough of them. Fresh is always best, but if you can't get them fresh, super foods (green powders made from fresh vegetables) will assure you of not missing out on important nutrients.

## Tip #3

### Probiotics

Probiotics refer to the friendly bacteria that live in the gastrointestinal tract. Meaning "pro-life," probiotics are the opposite of antibiotics. Probiotic supplements are most effective when taken daily as a preventive measure against illness.

## Tip #4

### Angstrom minerals

The body requires minerals for the composition of body fluids, the building of blood and bones, healthy nerve function, and muscle tone. The body's chemical balance depends on the levels of minerals in the body. If one level is out of balance, all the others are affected; this can cause other imbalances, and lead to illness. Angstrom minerals are so good for your healing because in angstrom form, they are so small that they get right into the bloodstream and do the job.

## Tip#5

*Chlorophyll*

**Wheatgrass and E-3 Live**

Chlorophyll is created in plants as a result of a conversion of the sun's energy. When we eat plants containing chlorophyll, this vital energy is transferred to us. In addition, the chlorophyll molecule is very similar to that of hemoglobin, the oxygen carrier in the blood. Leafy green vegetables are the best source of chlorophyll. Seaweed, algae and wheatgrass are other good sources.

## A POSITIVE WAY OF LIFE

The way you eat and think is helpful in curing yourself of IBD, but, still, to assure yourself of being cured, you want to approach life in a positive way always. Here are some tips that will help you do that:

## Tip #1

**Avoid negative people and situations.**

Stress of any kind can cause you to have problems with your IBD. Avoid these situations as much as possible. Stay positive. You either become like the people around you, or they become like you.

## Tip #2

**Let God into your life.**

Nothing can relieve stress more than letting God into your life. There is a certain path in life that we are all on. I believe getting IBD was part of the plan to shape me and make me the person I am today. Before I learned healthful eating, I didn't pay much attention to knowing God. My life was full of stress, worry, and no matter how much I had materially, I wasn't as happy as I knew I could be. That all changed when, after a set of circumstances, I couldn't ignore my spiritual need any longer. I let God into my life, and my life has changed. I believe this is the first and last step in the cure for IBD through getting healthy. Opening up my mind to God was the beginning, and it ended when I opened my heart to God. I am not suggesting that you must believe in God to be healthy and cured of IBD. It's not the only way. Many people have cured themselves without this step; but I am suggesting that there is no better way to get healthy and stay healthy. Why settle for anything less than the best? Please don't take my word for it. Go, and see for yourself. The best way to do this is to just start reading the best book in the world — the book with all the answers to everything: how to be healthy, how to stay happy and healthy, how to get the best investment in the world, etc. That book is the Bible. I meet so many people who say they don't believe in the Bible, but have never read it. How do you even know what it says unless you've read it? Once I read the Book of Daniel in the Bible, I saw how important it is to eat healthfully; and even more, how important it is to listen to God. There is a saying, "Ask, and you shall receive." Through prayer you can get cured of your IBD!

## Tip #3

**Relax.**

Slow down and enjoy life. When I was younger, I had a big sign on the wall in my room "Too fast to live, too young to die." I should have listened to it because I was sure living the fast life. Sleep and rest were not part of my list. I was always on the go, and it did catch up with me — I got IBD. Relaxation is one of the major keys to curing your IBD. Find time each day to relax. Sleeping and relaxing is healing, and whenever you avoid rest, you're avoiding healing. Get as much rest as you can.

## Tip #4

**Visualize.**

See inside your mind the person you want to become. Do you want to be healthy and cured of your illness? What's stopping you? How come some people can try everything I've suggested and not get cured? Because they never see themselves as cured. That's why. You must envision yourself as a healthy person, if you want to be a healthy person.

## Tip #5

**Believe.**

Trust in yourself; trust in God. Have faith. Never give up. You can make it. No matter how bad it seems, have faith that you will get cured. A setback is only a lesson, not a failure. Don't give up. Some of the most popular inventions in the world came from people who had many setbacks before they found what worked. The only people that fail are those who stop trying.

## Tip #6

**Be thankful.**

You will get what you pray for. Appreciate it, and it will continue to grow. What is better to be thankful for than your health? Nothing. There is no amount of money that can buy health. When you're not sick, you don't know what it is to feel and live with the misery of something like IBD, but once you've experienced it and get cured, being thankful is very easy and highly suggested.

## CONCLUSION

No matter how healthy you are, or how healthfully you eat, if you are not living your passion, it's going to be very hard to maintain a healthy body. Does everything you do make you happy all the time? When you get out of bed in the morning, are you happy and excited to get up and start you day? Do you look forward to going to work, or do you dread it? If you were to win the lottery tomorrow and had all the money you would ever need, would you still continue to live your life the way you do now? If you answer 'no,' then you are not living your true passion, and you're setting yourself up for a big fall. Curing yourself of a disease will not mean much if you're not living your passion.

### SPARK OR FIRE?

## Are you living your true desire?

We're all born with a spark inside us. It was once a fire, but has diminished to a spark after we've spent our time putting dirt into our bodies. The spark is still there waiting to be ignited. The way to add fuel back to the spark and rekindle the fire is to clean the mind, body and soul. Healing the body of disease is a good place to start, but we have to continue from there.

# Part Four

## Meal Planning

Many people, when first hearing about my cure for IBD, ask me to tell them what to eat and when to eat. We are not robots. No two people are in the same place at the same time, so it won't always be the same. The best meal plan I can suggest is to have set meal times.

I used to suggest that people not eat according to the clock. I used to say, "Eat only eat when you're hungry." I've changed my thinking about this after having come to the conclusion that most people don't always eat for the right reasons. They don't eat for true hunger, but out of habit hunger. They don't eat for nutrition, but for emotions. After seeing people time after time fail while eating whenever they're hungry, I've found that that is not the best way to eat. Eat by the clock. For example, pick a certain number of meals you're going to eat tomorrow and the times you're going to eat each meal. You don't have to have an exact type of food, but have a certain food category in that meal. For example: tomorrow I'm going to eat fruit at 9 a.m. for breakfast, at 12:30 p.m., I'm gong to have a big salad, and at 6 p.m., I'm going to have some nuts and a healthy raw "pizza" (there are many recipes for raw "pizza"). Eat at those times and no other. Some people like to do this and plan their meals for the whole week and some the night before. It doesn't matter, just know what is available, and base your choice on what's available. DO NOT EAT BETWEEN MEALS. Someone might say, "I'll just have a little snack, some fruits or something between meals." Your body doesn't know the difference between a full meal and a small snack. It has to work to digest it all. If you're hungry between meals, just have a fresh vegetable drink. That will hold you over untill the next meal. The key to doing this is when you do eat, make sure you eat enough, so you won't feel the need for food till your next meal. Now it all depends on how many meals you decide to eat each day. I suggest you even the meals out through-out the day. You don't have to start with three meals, but you will find in time that as you get healthier and make better food choic-es, you will want to eat less and less. Start by taking the number of times you now normally eat in a day, including snacks. Most people eat up to 7 to 10 times a day. Start with cutting that num-ber in half. So if you normally eat 3 meals a day and 3 snacks a day, that would be 6 times a day that you're eating. Start for about one month of only eating 3 times a day. You will see, in time, that you'll want to eat only twice a day. That's what I do, and it works great. Kiss emotional eating good-bye!

Now that you know when to plan your meals, what can you plan to include in your meals? The next part of this book will give you some great tasting, healthy recipes, but here are a few things to remember when it comes to your food choices:
Get the highest quality foods available: organic, fresh, ripe, fruits, vegetables, nuts and seeds. Do the best you can.

**Here are two important ways to improve your eating:**

A. - If you have the willpower, leave the bad stuff out. Health begins with what you leave out. Leave out the bad stuff.

Take all the things you know are bad for you, or bother your IBD, out of your diet. The common foods to avoid should be dairy, wheat, meat, bread, pasta, candy, cakes, cookies, soda, and coffee.

B - If you don't have the will power to leave out the bad stuff, make sure 75% of your diet is green leafy foods.

If you must eat the bad stuff, make sure, when you do eat,

that 75% of your meal has vegetables in it. Raw organic green leafy vegetables are the best – spinach, kale, etc. If you're going to drink soda and coffee, for every cup, add at least three green vegetable drinks. This will balance out the bad stuff you're eating, but the best choice is always to eat better by leaving out the bad stuff.

Once you have the meals scheduled ahead of time, including the foods you're going to eat, as I've suggested, the last thing to think about is combining your foods. Did you know there is an order of eating foods that can optimize your health? It's known as food combining.

# Part Five

## Recipes

Below, I've included two recipes you can use when you need help. As suggested, during an attack, these two recipes, adjusted to your personal taste, should be all that's taken. Additionally, you may drink green vegetable juices and take the whole live food supplements mentioned above.

### Almond Milk

1 cup soaked almonds
2 cups water
2 dates or 2 tablespoons honey
raw carob powder (optional) to taste

Blend all together and strain through a sprout bag or cheesecloth. Have a bowl underneath to catch the liquid. That liquid is the almond milk. Tastes great chilled.
You can use many different types of raw nuts other than almonds for a different taste.

### Blended Salad

There are so many different blended salads you can make. Start with this one as your base, and adjust it to your taste.

1 cucumber
1 tomato
1 stalk celery

75

juice of 1 lemon
handful of spinach
one avocado
a pinch of Celtic sea salt to taste.

No need to add water. Cut ingredients into small pieces and blend. As an option, you can use fennel instead of celery, or red pepper instead of cucumber. Or you can replace lemon juice with orange juice. The possibilities of adjusting a blended salad to your desired taste are endless

*Dr. David Klein*

# Part Six

## Resources

**Paul Nison**
PO Box 16156
West Palm Beach, FL 33416
917-407-2270
www.rawlife.com

For all your nutritional resources from enzymes, probiotics to green super food powders, plus many more, and books, videos and other items visit www.rawlife.com and click on the store. Paul Nison is also available for personal consultations.

**Dr. Fred Bisci**
125 Meadow Avenue
Staten Island, NY 10305
718-979-7950
www.fredbisci.com

Dr. Bisci does personal consultations. He has helped hundreds of people over the years by curing their ulcerative colitis and Crohn's disease. I suggest to anyone who is serious about healing any disease to follow the guidelines in this book. If you doubt any of the information, or would like to work with someone one on one, I suggest having a consultation with Dr. Bisci.

To order Fred Bisci products:
www.rawlife.com Click on the store